Bodybu

For Women:

The Ultimate Women's Fitness, Weight Training, Weight Lifting, Weight Loss Sports Program For The Ideal Female Body

By

Charles Maldonado

Table of Contents

Bodybuilding For Women: The Ultimate Women's
Fitness, Weight Training, Weight Lifting, Weight Loss
Sports Program For The Ideal Female Body

By Charles Maldonado

© Copyright 2015 Charles Maldonado

First Published, 2015

Printed in the United States of America

Introduction

Bodybuilding is not just about lifting weights and getting your body bulky. Bodybuilding is a sport that originated back in Europe during the 19th century which was more publicized by photography. There were pictures of body builders being sent to be used for promoting products so that people would buy them.

The sport of bodybuilding for women started in the 1960s, but the criteria for judging during the first contest for females were all based on the muscular development. This began with the U.S. Women's National Physique Championship back in 1978. This is the one that started it all for female bodybuilding.

From then on, bodybuilding for women has grown to be with proper standards that are more for the female form. A lot of women have learned to engage in bodybuilding and the hall of fame of female bodybuilders was first made in 1999.

This article will tell you what you need to know about bodybuilding especially that people think that it is more of a man's sport. There are specific types of food that you need to eat in order to support your bodybuilding routines and goals. There is no secret formula as to how you can achieve a body like that. It takes knowledge, determination, hard work, and not giving up. You need to push yourself harder so that you will progress through time and you will become satisfied with the results. You will also become stronger in performing daily activities and your endurance will build up. You also need to stay on track and check how you are progressing every day because that is one way you will be able to keep your motivation. You will see that the little efforts you are doing everyday are helping you become better and better. Don't be intimidated by what other people will say because body building is a journey you will start to take now and just like any other journey, you will also reach your destination as long as you stay disciplined in doing the things that need to be done and in following the principles that will also be mentioned in this article. After you have read this article, you will know more about body building and what are the foods you need to eat to support your training. You will also be given an example of a training plan that you can also choose to follow. It will also depend on your trainer if you can follow the training plan that will be provided here. You can use this article to help you in becoming a good body builder.

Chapter 1. Basic Principles of Body Building For Women

Principle 1 – 1 session should never exceed 60 minutes

One training session should never be more than 60 minutes. After 60 minutes has gone by, the muscle building hormone levels will start to drop. The carbohydrates that are present in your muscle cells and liver glycogen will be reduced. Glycogen is the one that fuels your muscles to become contracted. You will just end up doing useless weight training if you do it more than 60 minutes because you no longer have the hormones and muscle fuel to that are both needed to gain muscles. You will also end up overtraining your body if you go beyond 60 minutes. Your body will not be able to fully recover and you will lose both muscle mass and strength.

Principle 2 – When resting between sets, you should not exceed 90 seconds.

If you keep your resting time only 90 seconds or less, you will be able to perform better during the whole 60 minutes of your training and your cardiovascular health will also improve. It will also maximize the release of growth hormone which is very powerful for muscle building and fat burning. This interval of rest gives a volumizing effect to the muscles which means that the water will go inside the cells of the muscles making it look more toned and firm. This is not water retention.

Principle 3 – Weight training exercises

This should not be done for more than 2 consecutive days. This is something very important because other people tend to overlook this. Even if some people will be able to recover from 6 days in a week of weight training, it could still lead them to overtraining a particular muscle group or muscles. There are those who find it hard to recover from a training plan of 4 days a week. You should also avoid training the same muscle group for 2 days in a row because it takes 24 to 48 hours for muscle tissues to rebuild their torn tissues and recover from the training. Not giving your muscles to recover and rebuild will prevent muscle growth and strength to gain.

Principle 4 – Each set of weight training should have 6 to 15 repetitions

There are various reasons for this. First, it has been proven that when you do this range of repetitions you are able to maximize growth hormone for the muscles. This is very good because it builds muscles and your body fat will become less. Performing a lot of repetitions will get your blood pumping fast into the muscles which will give the muscles the nutrients they need to have a faster recovery and rebuild. When you do 6 to 15 repetitions, you are less prone to injury because you will only be using weight that you have total control of so that you can perform the repetitions that are required.

Principle 5 – You need to have progressive training

When you talk about progressive training, it means that you are doing more than the last session. You can do this by carrying a little more weight if you can exceed 15 repetitions in a particular movement. You should also know that it is not every session that you will increase the weight that you use to train. You can also do other forms of progressions like going a little over 60 minutes. The main goal of every training routine is that there should progression after some time so that there will be improvements when it comes to muscle definition and toning.

Principle 5 – Do varied training

This is important for promoting muscle gain and strength. This will also keep you from getting bored and it does not really mean that you would have to change your whole exercise routine. You can put variation in your training in other forms like doing a different kind of technique so that your muscles will become more stimulated. You can also change parameters, repetitions, rests in between sets, and you can create variation just by changing the grip you place on the bar so you can isolate other muscles. You will soon see that if you change up your routine and alternate them by doing 3 weeks of high-volume trainings and 3 weeks of training at a higher intensity, your body will gain maximum stimulus. If you did the same routines every day, you will experience staleness because the routine is only effective until your body will become used to it.

Principle 6 – Your form should be impeccable

Sometimes you want to perform weight training routines quickly to look impressive, but you are not aware that you are not being able to do the proper form because you want to show off. This can cause serious injuries to the muscle group that you are working on that might later need a surgery and you are not able to allow proper stimulation for that specific muscle group you are working on. This is because if you are not doing the correct form, other muscles will also start to work that will take away some focus on the muscle group that you are supposed to stimulate. This can slow down muscle growth and cause injury so you really need to pay attention.

Principle 7 – Aerobic exercise and other workouts done outside should be kept minimal

In order for you to get the maximum results when it comes to muscle mass, you need to minimize aerobics and other high-degree activities. This is because weight trainers have an extremely fast metabolism and if you do other high calorie burning activities, you will have a harder time gaining muscles because you will need a certain amount of calories to sustain the energy that you need during weight training and needed by muscle growth. Cardiovascular activity should also be limited to only 15 to 25 minutes for a couple times a week.

Principle 8 – It should be mostly composed of free weight exercises

Your training should mostly be composed of free weight exercises because they are the only ones that are able to give fast results by recruiting more muscles when you are performing the exercises. The body belongs to the three-dimensional universe. If you are working out on a machine, you are only allowing your body to work on a two-dimensional state because this will put a limit on the amount of muscle fibers that are supposed to be working. Machines are good for isolating muscles, but weight training should be dominated by dumbbells, and barbell exercises in which the body will move in a space like a dip, squat, and the pull-up.

Chapter 2. Foods You Must Eat For Bodybuilding

Mackerel – This is also under the tuna family, but this fish more omega-3 compared to tuna. This can help with the limiting chronic inflammation that can be caused by high intensity weight training. Mackerel has high levels of zinc which helps with building muscle. Zinc can also have a positive hormonal effect that is good for the thyroid glands to prevent decrease in hormones that is caused by intense training.

Beets- The nitrate that is found in beets can help with increasing vasodilation and your performance will also become better. A study shows that if you eat 2 medium beets 1 hour and 15 minutes prior to training, your performance will improve, the level of perceived exertion will be reduced, and it helps in decreasing the amount of oxygen that your body needs to perform the workout well.

Greek yogurt – This is produced by taking out excess liquid and carbohydrates from the regular yogurt. This is the reason why Greek yogurt contains more protein compared to regular yogurt. You still need to check the label before buying there are some that add gelling agents such as pectin and thickeners that can decrease the quality of Greek yogurt. The process that is done to take out the excess and carbohydrates in Greek yogurt creates highly-concentrated casein which is a milk protein that is slow-digesting which gives the body a stable increase of amino acid levels. Make sure that you will always get the plan one and stay away from the flavored ones because they can contain a lot of sugar.

Sardines – Tuna have a good reason to be popular, but if you want to get muscle-building power that is raw, sardines are better. They come in cans and ready to be eaten and this is not like tuna that is usually canned with water or vegetable oil. Sardines are usually found in extra-virgin olive oil. They also contain lesser mercury compared to albacore tuna. By just consuming 4 ounces of sardines, you are getting 1.8 grams of omega-3, but if you eat the same amount of tuna, you will only be getting 0.3 grams of omega-3. Omega-3 is good for the heart and it also has anti-inflammatory benefits that can also help with joint pain that is connected to high-volume training. Sardines also contain leucine which is an amino acid that is very effective because it becomes the catalyst for synthesizing protein.

Chocolate milk – This will be your best option after a training session if you don't have protein powder anymore. Chocolate milk has both casein proteins and whey. The extra sugar in chocolate milk will provide you with more carbohydrates which give more calories that are great for muscle building and also carbohydrates to boost recovery. A study shows that if you compare chocolate milk with the normal sports drink that has electrolytes and carbohydrates, it is better when it comes the muscle glycogen's resynthesizing. This stops the muscles from breaking down and pushes muscle growth because it helps the muscle-protein in synthesizing at a better level. There are also antioxidants found in cocoa which is present in chocolate milk. Antioxidants help with reducing oxidative, and muscle stress damage that is caused by intense training.

Almonds – Almonds have more protein and fiber compared to other nuts. If you take one shot glass full of almonds you are getting 6 grams of protein and 160 calories. They also contain a lot of vitamin e which is an alpha tocopherol. This is a very effective radical scavenger compared to the synthetic version that can be found in almost all supplements. Almond also contains a lot of vitamin b that helps in energizing metabolism which makes them perfect for anyone who wants gain mass with their diet. You will also get a body composition when you eat almonds to increase calories rather than carbohydrates.

Vinegar – When you need to shuttle nutrients to your muscles and not to your fat cells, vinegar will do that for you because that is a very important factor in lean muscle development. Studies show that when you add vinegar to a meal that contains a lot of carbohydrates, the carbohydrates will be stored as muscle glycogen. The vinegar becomes a trail guide that acts naturally to direct the carbohydrates to your muscles so that you will get enough energy and fuel preparing you for your next workout. This effect acts with food that contains denser carbohydrates like potatoes. You also don't need to consume much to get the benefits of vinegar. Your metabolism will become better with just 2 teaspoons of vinegar. You can add vinegar to the first meal that you will after a workout get the best glycogen-replenishing effects and add it again to the last meal you will have for the day that is packed with carbohydrates to get the best from the added calories, but at the same time keeping your insulin levels balanced and also how glucose is released in your body.

Lentils – These are packed with 3 of the most important nutrients you will need for your training. Lentils contain a lot of fiber, protein, and slow-digesting carbohydrates. A cup of lentils contains only 230 calories, with an impressive 18 grams of protein, and a total of 16 grams of fiber. When looking at lentils, you will see that they have 3 different varieties. They come in colors brown, red, and green with varying flavors depending on the color. Red lentils are faster to prepare because you will only 15 minutes to cook this, but the other 2 types require 30 to 45 minutes of cooking time.

Raspberries – This berry has various roles to play for muscle building. Digestive health is also improved so that your body will be able to fully get all the nutrients from any food that you eat. Among all berries, raspberry has the most fiber content. This contains 8 grams of fiber in one cup and keeping a high fiber diet is important for your body building diet. It helps in making your intestines work so that they will be in perfect shape. Raspberry is bright red in color because of the anthocyanin antioxidants. Anthocyanin will boost your brain to become more sensitive to leptin which is a very important for keeping your metabolic rate regulated and sensitive to insulin.

Quinoa- Quinoa is a grain that gives several advantages when it comes to nutritional and practicality compared to other forms of carbohydrates. Quinoa has unique components because it is not actually a grain. It is similar to rice and the quinoa plant that produces quinoa seeds are being harvested is similar to spinach. This is eaten to because of its benefits. If you take only one cup of quinoa, you are getting 8 grams of protein, 222 calories, twice the amount of fiber, zinc, and magnesium found in brown rice. Quinoa is one of the best muscle building foods because of the amino-acid profile it contains and also due to its low glycemic index which is only 53. This indicates that carbohydrates found in quinoa burns slower. This will give you an amount of calories that is well-sustained and also energy. Quinoa has all of the important amino acids compared to other carbohydrates. You only need 15 minutes to cook quinoa while brown rice needs 45 minutes cooking time.

Chapter 3. Bodybuilding Exercises For Women

Squats

Stand straight with your legs hip-width apart and keep your spine aligned, lower your butt down to the floor. Put force on your heels to push yourself back-up until you are able to stand straight again.

Do this for 15 repetitions.

Legs drops

Lay flat on your back and both of your legs extended straight up into the air with. Slowly lower both of your legs down to the floor, but do not let them touch the floor and keep your legs straight. You will that your lower back is popping off from the ground and by using your core muscles, move your feet back up into the air.

Do this for 10 repetitions.

Push ups

Starting in a plank position and keeping your spine straight. Put your arms under your, but the space between them should be slightly wider than your shoulders. Start to lower your body down, but do not let it touch the floor completely. Keep your spine straight and do not raise your butt. Push yourself back up.

If you are a beginner, you can lower your knees to the floor for more support but this will give less resistance to your core and arms.

Do this for 20 repetitions.

Chapter 4. Body Building Training Plan

For weeks 1, 2, and 3

Monday - You need to do 5 minutes of light cardio as your warm-up. This could be a 5-minute walk or light jog on a treadmill.

Squats

Do 5 repetitions as your warm-up set

Then do 5 sets of squats with 5 repetitions

Dead lifts

Do 5 repetitions as your warm-up set

Do 5 sets of dead lifts with 5 repetitions

Standing calf raise

Do 5 sets of 10 repetitions

Sit-ups in incline

Do 3 sets with 10 to 20 repetitions

Tuesday- Start again with 5 minutes of light cardio as your warm up. This could be on a stationary bike or a treadmill with low intensity.

Incline barbell bench press

Do 3 repetitions first as your warm-up

Do 5 sets of incline barbell bench press with 5 repetitions

Seated dumbbell shoulder press

5 sets of seated dumbbell shoulder press with 8 repetitions

 Bicep cable curls

5 sets of bicep cable curls with the 10 repetitions

Tricep push down

5 sets of tricep push downs with 10 repetitions

Dumbbell lateral raises

3 sets of dumbbell lateral raises with 10 to 15 repetitions

Thursday – 5 minutes of light cardio warm up.

Leg press

Do a couple as your warm-up

Do 4 sets of leg press with 15 repetitions

Leg curls

Do 4 sets of leg curls with 15 repetitions

Wide grip pull down

Do 4 sets of wide grip pull with for 15 repetitions

Hyper extensions

Do 4 sets of hyperextensions with 10 repetitions

Ab crunches

Do 4 sets of ab crunches with 15 repetitions

Friday – Start with a 5-minute light cardio as your warm-up

Incline dumbbell bench press

Do 2 repetitions as your warm-up set

Do 4 sets of dumbbell bench press with 10 repetitions

Dumbbell side lateral raises

Do 4 sets of dumbbell side lateral raises with 10 repetitions

Bicep dumbbell curls

Do 4 sets of bicep dumbbell curls with 12 repetitions

Tricep push downs

Do 4 sets of tricep push downs with 12 repetitions

Barbell upright rows

Do 3 sets of barbell upright rows with 15 repetitions

Monday – 5 minutes cardio warm-up (cardio can also be walking on a treadmill or a light jog)

Bent over barbell rows

Do 3 repetitions as your warm-up set

Do 5 sets of bent over barbell rows with 8 repetitions

Barbell shoulder shrugs

Do 5 sets of barbell shoulder shrugs with 10 repetitions

Leg extensions

Do 5 sets of leg extensions with 10 repetitions

Leg curls

Do 5 sets of leg curls with 10 repetitions

Seated calf raise

Do 5 sets of seated calf raise with 10 repetitions

Incline sit-ups

Do 5 sets of incline sit-ups with 10 repetitions

Tuesday – Start with 5 minutes of light cardio as your warm up

Decline barbell bench press

Do a few repetitions first as your warm-up

Do 5 sets of decliner barbell bench press with 5 repetitions

Seated barbell shoulder press

Do 5 sets of barbell shoulder press with 8 repetitions

Preacher barbell curls

Do 5 sets of preacher barbell curls with 10 repetitions

Lying tricep extension

Do 5 sets of lying tricep extensions with 10 repetitions

Cable upright rows

Do 3 sets of cable upright rows with 15 repetitions

Thursday – Start with 5 minutes of light cardio

Hack squat

Do a few repetitions as your warm-up

Do 4 sets of hack squat with 15 repetitions

Stiff leg dead lifts

Do 4 sets of stiff leg dead lifts with 15 repetitions

Seated cable rows

Do 4 sets of seated cable rows with 15 repetitions

Leg raises

Do 4 sets of leg raises with 12 repetitions

Crunches

Do 4 sets of crunches with 25 or more repetitions

Friday – Start with 5 minutes of light cardio

Flat dumbbell bench press

Do a few repetitions as your warm-up

Do 4 sets of flat dumbbell bench press with 10 repetitions

Dumbbell front lateral raises

Do 4 sets of dumbbell front lateral raises with 10 repetitions

Bicep barbell curls

Do 4 sets of bicep barbell curls with 12 repetitions

Tricep push downs

Do 4 sets of tricep push downs with 12 repetitions

Close grip pull down

Do 4 sets of close grip pull down with 15 repetitions

Monday – 5 minutes of soft cardio to warm you up

Squats

Do 6 repetitions first as your warm-up

Do 5 sets of squats with 5 repetitions

Partial dead lifts

Do a few repetitions first as your warm up

Do sets of partial dead lifts with 5 repetitions

Chin ups

4 sets of chin ups with as many repetitions as you can

Pull down ab crunches

Do 5 sets of pull down ab crunches with 10 repetitions

Leg raises

Do 5 sets of leg raises with 5 repetitions

Tuesday – Do 5 minutes of soft cardio as your warm-up

Flat barbell bench press

Do a few first as your warm-up

Do 5 sets of flat barbell bench press with 5 repetitions

Bent over dumbbell lateral raises

Do 4 sets of bent over dumbbell lateral raises with 10 repetitions

Dumbbell front lateral raises

Do 4 sets of dumbbell front lateral raises with 10 repetitions

Bicep cable curls

Do 5 sets of bicep cable curl with 10 repetitions

Tricep push downs

Do 5 sets of tricep push downs with 10 repetitions

Thursday – Start with 5 minutes of soft cardio

Hack squat

Do a few first to warm you up

Do five sets of hack squats with 10 repetitions

Leg press

Do four sets of leg press with 15 repetitions

Chest supported rows

Do four sets of chest supported rows with 10 repetitions

Hyper extensions

Do four sets of hyper extensions with 10 repetitions

Pull down ab crunches

Do four sets of pull down ab crunches with 10 repetitions

Friday – Start with 5 min of soft cardio

Stability ball dumbbell bench press

Do a few first for warm up

Do four sets of stability ball dumbbell bench press with 10 repetitions

Stability ball sitting dumbbell shoulder press

Do four sets of stability ball dumbbell shoulder press with 10 repetitions

Bar bicep curls

Do four sets of bar bicep curls with 12 repetitions

Overhead dumbbell extensions with one arm

Do four sets of overhead dumbbell extensions with one arm for 12 repetitions

One arm dumbbell rows

Do 3 sets of one arm dumbbell rows with 15 repetitions

Monday - Start with 5 minutes of soft cardio for warm up

Leg press

Do a few first as warm up

Do 5 sets of leg press with 5 repetitions

Stiff leg dead lifts

Do a few first as warm up

Do 5 sets of stiff leg dead lifts with 5 reps

Wide grip pull downs

Do four sets of wide grip pull downs with 10 repetitions

Incline sit ups

Do 5 sets of incline sit ups with 15 repetitions

Leg raises

Do 5 sets of leg raises with 15 repetitions

Tuesday – Do 5 minutes of soft cardio as warm up

Dips

Do a few first as warm up

Do 5 sets of dips with 5 repetitions

Chin ups

Do four sets with as many repetitions that you can do

Side lateral raises

Do four sets of side lateral raises with 10 repetitions

Seated barbell shoulder press

Do four sets of seated barbell shoulder press with 10 repetitions

Tricep push downs

Do 5 sets of tricep push downs with 10 repetitions

Bicep dumbbell preacher curls

Do 5 sets of bicep dumbbell preacher curls with 10 repetitions

Thursday – Start with 5 minutes of soft cardio as warm up

Squats

Do four sets of squats with 15 repetitions

Leg curls

Do four sets of leg curls with 15 repetitions

Leg extensions

Do four sets of leg extensions with 15 repetitions

Seated cable rows

Do four sets of seated cable rows with 10 repetitions

Standing calf raise

Do four sets of standing calf raise with 10 repetitions

Pull down ab crunches

Do four sets of pull down ab crunches with 15 repetitions

Friday – Do 5 min of soft cardio as warm up

Elevated feet stability ball push up

Do four sets with as many as you can do

Seated dumbbell shoulder press

Do four sets of seated dumbbell shoulder with 10 repetitions

One arm dumbbell curls

Do four sets of one arm dumbbell curls with 12 repetitions

Overhead dumbbell extension with one arm

Do four sets of overhead dumbbell extensions with one are with 12 repetitions

Close grip pull downs

Do four sets of close grip pull downs with 15 repetitions

How long should one session be?

Weight training sessions should never exceed 60 minutes to avoid overtraining and your muscle building hormones no longer work beyond 60 minutes so any workout done beyond 60 minutes would become useless. To know how many times you should workout in a week, follow the training plan given.

Conclusion

Body building is no longer for men and it is also becoming a popular sport for women. It started in 1978 for women, but it was not as popular as it is today. If you want to get started with bodybuilding, consider all of the tips, principle, foods, and training plan mentioned in this article so you can have a better head start on the steps that you need to take.

Thank You Page

I want to personally thank you for reading my book. I hope you found information in this book useful and I would be very grateful if you could leave your honest review about this book. I certainly want to thank you in advance for doing this.

If you have the time, you can check my other books too.

Lightning Source UK Ltd.
Milton Keynes UK
UKHW022005260922
409473UK00006B/388